Intermittent Fasting Simplified
Look Better, Live Longer

By Alexander Rioux

Foreword

To those along the journey of self-improvement. There is no nobler pursuit. To folks in plateaus, rough patches, and dire situations. To those inches from surrender.
Never give up, for life.

A.Rioux

Table of Contents

Introduction

As a young man with a relentless desire to build a lean and powerful physique, I had tried many of the traditional dieting methods for fat loss and muscle gain. With each passing attempt, my motivation waned further. After hitting failure after failure; plateau after plateau; I began to question my own fortitude. 'How would I ever be able to accomplish anything in my life if I can't even take control of my own diet and physicality?' was the conversation that often played out in my mind. The ever-so-common six small meals per day routine left me feeling like a fawn as I grazed in the grass all day. Never truly satisfying my hunger, and always left wanting for the next meal coming in just a few hours. After a few months it was clear that this method of dieting required far more effort than it was worth. If you're a busy individual like most of us in this day and age- planning, preparing, and carrying a full day's worth of food at all times ranges from being a hassle to a an absolute nightmare. I then moved into the household standard low carb diet that rose to prominence through Dr. Atkins in 1972. Who hasn't tried low-carbing at some point, right? It seems simple. The instructions are straight-forward. On this diet, the lack of energy I felt around the clock was near debilitating. The body needs carbohydrates to convert into glucose. Our bodies use this glucose as fuel for our brains, livers, among many other organs and processes. It is akin to gasoline in our human fuel tank. After a few weeks dieting this way, I began to seek alternatives once again. I bounced around between countless other styles of dieting. The main issue I found with typical diets is that they require some level of *deprivation* and *restriction* as an essential facet of their framework. Of course, any endeavor that one finds meaningful will require some form of deprivation and restriction during the journey. I don't believe any Ph.D. student has published a thesis without a considerable amount of restriction on their schedule during the writing process. Nor do I believe any addict has freed themselves of addiction without having to deprive themselves of substances at many points along the way. These threads are quite commonplace even in our day-to-day lives as parents, colleagues, and peers. We must restrict our free leisure time in order to maintain the responsibilities of our career and working lives. We must deprive ourselves of distraction to maintain focus on tasks. These happen on a small scale (both consciously and unconsciously) every single day. They are often necessary evils in simply getting things done. However, humans have a tendency to over complicate things. This tends to happen very often with dieting, fitness, and health. I started to wonder if this was true in my case. If the needless deprivation and restriction I was employing in my diets was a help or a hinderance. Having been this far along in my quest, I was well acquainted with these threads. I welcomed them. I was prepared to work hard and make the necessary sacrifices- it's what I signed up for after all. About two years into this journey however, I began feeling the adverse mental effects of being so deprived for so long. The conversation in my head changed from a jovial and tenacious can-do attitude to a defeated and self-deprecating tenor. I knew I wasn't just going to give up. I also knew that the methods I had been utilizing were proving less and less fruitful as time went on. A pragmatic individual, I began to ask myself- "Is this much sacrifice actually required of me?".

I began to wonder if I was making the right type of sacrifices.

Common industry advice always leans toward *doing more.* Need to lose those last 15 pounds? Eliminate **more** starch and processed food from your diet. Further **restrict** your caloric intake. Perform **more** aerobic exercise. Increase the intensity of your resistance training sessions. This is also partially a symptom of the Western mindset. Of course, there is a ceiling on how far you can go before physically burning out, just as there is a ceiling on how long your brain can work before it requires rest and recovery. Often times, we believe we have reached our limit physically long before it even happens. The mind games we play with ourselves can wreak havoc on our outlooks and hinder our progress. Upon recognizing this, I looked to science for an answer. An answer to solve the mental game, understanding that the battles we wage in our minds are ultimately the most crucial battles we fight on route to achieving what we set out to.

Cue the forum section of *bodybuilding.com*. I came across an insightful article on the relatively new concept of intermittent fasting. It seemed to provide solutions to many of the problems I faced. It appeared to answer many questions that lingered in the fitness world surrounding weight loss and diet structure. Initially, I was pessimistic. This went against everything I had learned, seen, and been taught regarding weight loss and muscle gain. But I had to be sure. I went about my due diligence and read many excerpts from acclaimed scientific journals, encyclopedias, and publications. The data was there. The research was solid. The theses were proven. I made the decision to give it a go. I ate a large dinner one evening and abstained from consuming calories until lunch the next day. I was, as they say, "off to the races". Fast forward eight years to today. I reached my goal of 195lbs at 8% bodyfat (5'11) somewhere around the year 2017 utilizing intermittent fasting principles throughout the whole journey. I've been able to maintain this condition 365 days per year, every year, while being able to enjoy life as it is meant to be enjoyed. No living inside a box gym and far from hauling a large bag of Tupperware containers everywhere. I've been able to make steady increases in strength and athleticism over this period. Although my original goal was vanity-based, I couldn't help but notice the additional health benefits from the process. I was sick less often. Moreover, whenever I did fall ill, my recovery was dramatically shorter than it had been prior to following IF. My skin looked noticeably more clear and vibrant. My mental ability to index, recall, and recite information was enhanced. My cognition became sharper. Once again, my curiosity peaked. What I then uncovered about the physiological of intermittent fasting had me hooked- eager to refine my methods and achieve a better quality of life. These findings are the basis of the book.

I believe all people have the tools required to undergo the journey to their best self. Intelligence, grit, perseverance. Fortitude, diligence, consistency. What most are lacking is a thorough plan, a framework through which one can employ these efforts. A sustainable plan- one that allows the living of a full and enriched life as well- provides the best odds for being successful in an endeavour long term. This is why I wrote *Intermittent Fasting Simplified: Look Better, Live Longer.* While I cannot guarantee your physical results, I can guarantee that these principles are solid. They are born in, and backed by science. They work when abided by, without fail. Join me as we dive deep into the science of this method and provide insight into how it can be incorporated into your life with relative ease. This is not a book of secrets, nor magic potions. It is not a set of strict guidelines that you 'must' follow. Rather, it is a culmination of research and practical application, studied over nearly a decade. You will not be told what to do. You will not be instructed. In contrast, you will be presented with 50+ studies worth of information, digested and consolidated into one guide. You will be shown the tactics with the option to make your own decisions based on where your life is at and where you'd like it to be. You'll be offered viable and practical solutions to problems that many face in their pursuit of health and happiness. Last of all (and certainly not least) you'll finally be on your way to the fit, healthy, wonderful physique you've always knew you deserved. Without further ado, let's get to it.

The only thing you stand to lose, is weight.

What is Intermittent Fasting?

Intermittent fasting (or "IF") is an eating pattern that involves cycling between distinct periods of feeding and fasting. These periods are defined by, and specific to each individual according to their lifestyle and overall goals. Typically, the fasting window is at least twice as long in duration as the feeding window. For example, a person looking to use an 8-hour feeding window will have a 16-hour fasting window. Another individual who can better fit a 6-hour feeding window will have an even longer fasting period at 18 hours. There are a specific set of physiological processes that occur as a result of these windows. They form the benefits that are obtained as a result of following IF. The cognitive enhancement, increased life expectancy, and propensity for weight loss and muscle gain are just a few of these. We will look much deeper into the science of these during later chapters. For those reasons and many more, IF is a popular health and fitness trend today. It has really come into the forefront of the health and fitness community during the late 2010's. This science is anything but new, however. The practice and study of fasting have been around for centuries. One major proponent of fasting as a healing method was Hippocrates, the ancient Greek philosopher whose works are still widely quoted and referenced today. Men and women of his time operated on the belief that fasting was an 'internal physician' that would alert someone that health issues were present. It was initially believed that fasting was the standard for treating all sorts of illnesses and maladies. Fasting has remained a prominent part of many Eastern and old world cultures throughout the millennia. Its benefits are too great to ignore.

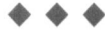

Typical diets purported in the Western world focus solely on the *consumption* of food. They center themselves around feeding without stressing an understanding of what happens biologically when we abstain from doing so. Things like what type of foods to eat, the best times to consume them, and in which quantities are taught to us unambiguously from a young age. I'm sure most remember health classes in primary school where the teacher would bring out the food pyramid chart and begin talking about the various food groups. Meat and poultry, fruits and vegetables, dairy and grains. We're taught of serving sizes, recommended amounts, and daily allowances. It's understood that eating a healthy, balanced diet and exercising regularly will keep the unwanted weight off and have you at your best. That is much easier said than done, especially in the fast-paced times we live in today. Time constraints and available food options are typically the bottlenecks of this operation. Counting calories and cooking multiple times per day aren't often feasible nowadays. The key difference with IF is the strategic planning of longer fasting periods that allow us to tap into some of the major health and weight loss benefits associated with said abstinence. These will be discussed at length in the Benefits chapter. In short, the body undergoes a few significant biological processes when faced with the daily internal stress of fasting. Overall, these result in increased weight loss, improved insulin response, and anti-aging effects. This happens while you're still able to enjoy the foods you love in fulfilling quantities every single day. Trust me. I'm not making this up!

Intermittent fasting is ideal for anyone who will not endure complications greater than the benefits provided by adhering to the method. There are no prerequisites that make any one person a better candidate for using this method, no one group of people who stand to benefit more than others. However, due to the nature of the feeding/ fasting cycles and the effects they have on the body, it is imperative that you consult your medical professional before beginning to fast in this manner. Some conditions or genetic precursors may not allow affected individuals to adopt these principles successfully. An example may be those afflicted with diabetes (Type I or II). Studies have shown that these individuals do not respond as positively to fasting as they would on a typical restricted-calorie diet. Research shows that the most optimal solution for this group is to focus more on aggregate carbohydrate consumption at a sustained pace. In addition, test subjects were frequently required to have their blood glucose levels tested and recorded by medical staff- reiterating the above point with regards to consulting a medical doctor. This advice is paramount for intermittent fasting, yet remains true when beginning any sort of diet, exercise, or supplement regime. Health and medical professionals have studied and trained for a substantial amount of time in order to be able to assess and treat our bodies. It is important to seek their opinions as they have access to data and instruments that we do not, to provide answers that we cannot derive on our own. Regular check-ups are recommended for anyone at any stage, on any program, in any part of the world. With that being said, once you've sought a professionals' opinion and received the green light to dive into the wonderful world of fasting, let's get you there.Our next few chapters will take a look at the overarching objectives of intermittent fasting to gain insight into exactly what processes occur and why the method is effective as a result. Once we've got a grasp on the overall concept, we will be talking about how to apply it. Last, the specifics on how to implement IF into your life individually.

The Main Benefits of IF

Now that we have an idea of what this whole fasting thing entails, let's dive into its benefits. It seems every other day I come across a new benefit proven through scientific study. Other times, further study will indicate that an already-known benefit has a much greater scope than initally thought. There are a vast amount of personal benefits one may find when following this method. For example, more free time at home with your family may be something you get to experience. For others, they may appreciate being able to eat until full. There are all sorts of reported benefits from IF proponents. For the purpose of this book, I try to avoid speculation, sticking to verified and studied concepts for the sake of objectivity. With this being said, I could quite easily write a hundred pages on the benefits that I personally have come across in my years of adopting the method. Most of these will be addressed at the relevant points in the book. I've compiled the 5 major benefits that science has uncovered thus far. No matter your physique goal, these benefits are made possible for everyone by fasting. Let's get into it.

Autophagy

Increased autophagy is an incredible benefit to be obtained from intermittent fasting. In my opinion, it's the most valuable benefit available due to its profound effects on overall health. Autophagy, by definition, is the natural, regulated mechanism of the cell that disassembles unnecessary or dysfunctional components. It allows the orderly degradation and recycling of cellular components. It was the subject of the 2016 Nobel Prize, awarded to a Japanese doctor named Yoshinori Ohsum. He discovered the autophagy mechanism and how it is triggered by stress and fasting.

In fact, autophagy is so beneficial that it's now being called a "key in preventing diseases such as cancer, neuro-degeneration, cardiomyopathy, diabetes, liver disease, autoimmune diseases and infections" (as per the U.S. National Institute of Health). Before discussing its immense benefits, let's take a simpler look at what autophagy is to understand this highly complex biological process. In layman's terms, autophagy is the process of purging waste from the body and remodeling the cells to function more efficiently. The body naturally performs this cleansing to a degree, no matter how often you fast (if at all). This cycle of waste and regeneration is seen across many different biological systems of the body. However, there is a remarkable difference in the efficacy of this process when we introduce consistent daily fasts. Even more so when paired with a steady exercise routine. Consider the following list of benefits stemming from autophagy.

- *Regulating functions of cells' mitochondria, which help produce energy but can be damaged by oxidative stress*
- *Clearing damaged endoplasmic reticulum and peroxisomes*

- *Protecting the nervous system and encouraging growth of brain and nerve cells. Autophagy seems to improve cognitive function, brain structure and neuroplasticity.*
- *Supporting growth of heart cells and protecting against heart disease*
- *Enhancing the immune system by eliminating intracellular pathogens*
- *Defending against misfolded, toxic proteins that contribute to a number of amyloid diseases*
- *Protecting stability of DNA*
- *Preventing damage to healthy tissues and organs (known as necrosis)*
- *Recycling damaged proteins, organelles and aggregates*

To sum it up, autophagy has been proven to have dramatic anti-aging and longevity effects. It entices your body to repair, recycle, and regenerate vital cells that otherwise may lead to inflammatory illnesses or other diseases if dormant in the body too long. Currently underway are studies being performed to determine how strong the link is between fasting, autophagy, and reduction of cancerous cells in affected patients. While science is still coming to terms with the true scope of its effectiveness, it has been validated through study after study to provide the afore-mentioned benefits and more.

Gotta love fasting!

Improved Insulin Response

Another major benefit that IF provides is improving in-sulin response. Much like its effects on autophagy, these benefits can't be observed by the naked eye. Nonetheless, they are extremely powerful. The basic role of insulin in the body is to allow for conversion of sugar into energy (glucose), as well as regulation of blood sugar levels to avoid a surplus (hyperglycemia) or a deficit (hypoglycemia). Taken a step further, regularly operating in a hyperglycemic state is what's responsible for the epidemic of Type-II diabetes in the United States. It is estimated that 1 in 10 Americans have diabetes, with 90-95% of cases being Type-II. I'm sure we all know someone afflicted with this illness. It can be quite difficult to deal with, especially when co-morbidities are present. Type-I is hereditary, but Type-II is largely result of habit. So what can we do to improve these habits?

Fasting is the most efficient and consistent strategy to decrease insulin levels. This was first noted decades ago, and widely accepted as true. It is really quite simple. All foods raise insulin, so the most effective method of reducing insulin is to avoid all foods. Blood glucose levels remain normal, as the body begins to switch over to burning fat for energy. This effect is seen with fasting periods as short as 24-36 hours. Longer duration fasts reduce insulin even more dramatically.Regular fasting, in addition to lowering insulin levels, has also been shown to improve insulin sensitivity significantly. This is the missing link in the weight loss puzzle. Most diets reduce highly insulin-secreting foods, but do not address the insulin resistance issue. Weight is initially lost, but insulin resistance keeps insulin levels and Body Set Weight high. Fasting is an efficient method of reducing insulin resistance. Lowering insulin rids the body of excess salt and water. Cosmetically, this creates a more tighter and leaner look on our frame. Within the body, insulin causes salt and water retention in the kidney. Atkins-style diets often cause diuresis, the loss of excess water, leading to the contention that much of the initial weight loss is water. While true, diuresis is beneficial in reducing bloating, and feeling 'lighter'. Some may also note a slightly lower blood pressure. Fasting has been noted to have a period of rapid weight loss initially, stemming mostly from this process.

Adrenalin & Adrenal Glands

This is really quite interesting. Fasting, but not low-calorie diets results in numerous hormonal adaptations that all appear to be highly beneficial on many levels. In essence, fasting transitions the body from burning sugar to burning fat. Resting metabolism is not decreased as many would assume, but instead increased. We are, effectively, feeding our bodies through our own fat. We are 'eating' our own fat. This makes total sense. Fat, in essence is stored food. In fact, studies show that the epinephrine (adrenalin) induced fat burning does not depend upon lowering blood sugar. Recall our previous discussion of How Insulin Works. Fat is food stored away in the long term, like money in the bank. Short term food is stored as glycogen, like money in the wallet. The problem we have, is how to access the money in the bank. As our wallet depletes, we become nervous and go out to fill it again. This prevents us from getting access to money in the bank. Fat is stored away in the 'bank'. As our glycogen 'wallet' depletes, we get hungry and want to eat. That makes us hungry, despite the fact that there is more than enough 'food' stored as fat in the 'bank'. How do we get to that fat to burn it? Fasting provides an easy way in.

Greater Focus and Concentration

This benefit piggybacks onto the previous one in the sense of freeing mental space to redirect it towards your other pursuits in life. The deeper benefit is the great improvement in focus during the fasting window. In mammals, mental activity increases when hungry and decreases with satiation. We have all experienced this as 'food coma'. Think about that large Thanksgiving turkey and pumpkin pie. After that huge meal, are we mentally sharp as a tack? Or dull as a concrete block? How about the opposite? Think about a time that you were really hungry. Were you tired and slothful? I doubt it. Your senses were probably hyper-alert and you were mentally sharp as a needle. The idea that food make you concentrate better is entirely incorrect. There is a large survival advantage to animals that are cognitively sharp, as well as physically agile during times of food scarcity.

A 1997 study showed that Although glucose levels were lowered following food deprivation (fasting), there was no significant detrimental effect of food deprivation on task performance. However, improved recognition memory processing times were associated with deprivation. Incentive motivation was associated with faster simple reaction times and higher diastolic blood pressure. There were no significant relationships between glucose levels and task performance, further supporting the hypothesis that the brain is relatively invulnerable to short food deprivation. In fact, studies show that cognitive function improved in fasting individuals, most notably during the fast itself. Initially, as you reset your feeding clock, you may experience hunger pangs or cravings during this time. In some cases, they may be strong enough to detract your focus initially. This is understandable as your body is used to receiving nutrition around the clock, at various times of the day. Switching to a structured style of eating will take your body some time to get accustomed to. Once this stage is reached, however, the immense benefits of fasting become evident.

More Free Time

This was a benefit I observed right away. I personally began implementing intermittent fasting into my routine after following a six meals per day regime. Whether a meal was cooked at home from scratch, or a readily consumable snack, much thought had to have gone into scheduling the feedings of the day. After the thought came the calculations and planning. Can I afford to add a tablespoon of dressing to my salad this evening?

Following that, I would procure the necessary meals to fill my six slots. Between the decision making, calorie calculation, and preparation times, I found myself spending an awful lot of a precious resource planning something that shouldn't be so complicated. The preoccupation with food alone exhausted my brain day after day after day. This is a more extreme example- common habit in Western society is to consume the standard three meals per day. When consuming breakfast in the morning, you are feeding all day. From your initial meal until your final bite, you must be equally conscious of what you are eating and equally focused on what remains available for the day. This is not to say that the practice of nutrient calculation and planning are thrown out the window. They are just as important under intermittent fasting as they are under any other umbrella of dieting style. Planning two or three meals is objectively easier than four to six. Occupying your mind with your diet is far more manageable when done for 8 hours a day as opposed to 16. Your choices when delegating 2,000 calories may be far more liberal when working within a half-day window as opposed to an entire one. Once you have found your rhythm, your flow, with regards to eating this way- things become automatic. Your body understands what to eat and when, while your mind understands the nutrient profiles of the foods you eat over time. You'll save ample tangible time and free up immense intangible focus. Trust me.

The Fasting Window

We will now look at the fasting window in a little more detail. It is after all, where the majority of the magic happens regarding increased fat burning, lean mass retention, and disease prevention. It is important to note the distinction between a caloric fast and an abstinence fast. In an abstinence fast, you abstain from consuming anything whatsoever- even water. A good example of this would be the practice of Ramadan, adhered to by Muslims worldwide. During this period, the adherents abstain from consuming any food or water while the sun is visible. From sun up in the morning, to sun down in the evening, a Muslim may consume nothing. In addition, Muslims must refrain from sexual behaviours and otherwise distasteful mannerisms during the *sawm* period. This practice is derived from religious customs and seeks to achieve different goals than we have set out to here. The practice of Ramadan has great spiritual implications and guides the follower to practice restraint- symbolic of understanding God's gifts and improving compassion for the deprived.

When fasting for the purposes outlined in this book, the requirements are much more relaxed (enjoy all the sex you please... it's great cardio). Please appreciate that our goal when fasting is to activate the hormonal responses that contribute to fat burning, muscle gain, and overall regulation of physiological processes. Although you may find this experience to be spiritual and enlightening, these are not bonafide requirements of making some serious progress in achieving a healthy mind and high-performance physique. You may be asking "what is permitted during the fast"? The goal here is to drink only water throughout the fast. This ensures that no trace calories are consumed, and the fasted state is maintained until the next feeding window. Drinks that bear no calories will have the same (negligible) effects as water. Some household examples include black tea and black coffee. They must be taken in a manner free of calories, meaning no added sugar or dairy. There are also a bevy of different zero calorie drinks on the market that are suitable for consumption in this circumstance. **Diet Coke, Coke Zero, Pepsi Max** are some common soft drink (carbonated) beverages available to fit this bill.

Taken a step further, there are also an increasingly large number of zero calorie energy drinks coming to the market. These include, but are not limited to, **Monster Zero, Red Bull Zero, and Rockstar Zero.**

The body does provide a slight bit of lee-way when following this method. One commonly held belief is that consuming < 30cal during this period will have little to no effect on maintaining a fasted state. Some examples of this include a splash of milk in your tea or coffee for taste, or some BCAA's with a minute calorie count. Be careful- the body will return to its baseline level of autophagy once it metabolizes protein of any kind. Although the calories consumed are widely believed to be within the acceptable threshold, the fact that they contain proteins will disrupt this process specifically. If your main goal is to attain the anti-aging effects of fasting, I would forego this addition. Initially, as your body accustoms itself to going through an extra 8 hours of fasted time, you will notice hunger pangs every once in a while. These may last anywhere from a few days to a few weeks. Try to remember that this is a result of the changes in hormones, and less a matter of your body physically requiring sustenance. So long as you are consuming the necessary macronutrients to sustain your activity level, this is quite literally all in your head. To expand this point, we will take a brief look at *leptin* and *ghrelin*, two major hormones that regulate appetite and hunger.

Leptin tells your brain that you have enough energy stored in your fat cells to engage in normal, relatively expensive metabolic processes. In other words, when leptin levels are at a certain threshold - your brain senses that you have energy sufficiency, which means you can burn energy at a normal rate, eat food at a normal amount, engage in exercise at a normal rate, and you can engage in expensive processes, like puberty and pregnancy.

Ghrelin is the hormone produced within the stomach that

serves to increase your appetite and regulate your body weight. These two hormones, while opposite in nature, create a sort of 'checks and balances' system between them that ensures your body is receiving adequate nutritional supply in order to operate. Many studies have shown leptin levels decreased significantly in those who were practicing time-restricted feeding (IF), but there was no negative effect on energy expenditure. In addition, participants report substantially less hunger pangs than their control group counterparts, following a traditional feeding style.

The long and short of it is that after acclimating your circadian rhythm to the two distinct windows, your body will go through less spikes in hunger and energy than following a traditional method of consumption. This is particularly positive for those who struggle with giving into dietary temptations. Out of mind, out of stomach (my keen adaptation on the classic 'out of sight, out of mind'). All the while, you will be experiencing energy and fat loss you never thought possible. When it becomes time to feed, the body is replenished, its stores are refilled, and it is properly prepared for yet another day.

The Feeding Window

Now's the part we've all been waiting for. It's time to eat. The feeding window is the period of time in the day at which you consume all of your daily caloric requirements. It is the net time remaining when subtracting the duration of your fasting period from the total time available in the day. Given the fact that the entirety of your meals are consumed within this window, it is important to choose a period of time that is comfortable for your lifestyle and schedule. With that being said, you will need to strike a balance between your desired time for fasting and your desired time for feeding. After all, there are only 24 hours in the day. Some common feeding window durations are shown below along with their implied fasting times.

Feeding Window	Fasting Window
10 hours	14 hours
8 hours	16 hours
6 hours	18 hours
4 hours	20 hours

The most common ratio is 8:16. This means eating your TDEE within 8 hours and consuming no calories for 16. Mathematically this breaks the day into thirds. As most people sleep for 8 hours of the day, this schedule would have you sleeping, fasting, and feeding for equal amounts of time in the day assuming 8 hours of sleep are had at night. In contrast to the increased benefits from a longer fasting period, science has yet to come up with an answer to optimal feeding times. No correlation has been found between greater results and longer/shorter feeding times. This is generally believed to be because each individual's metabolism differs greatly. As far as experimental studies go, it proves difficult to determine the *exact* exit of the fed state and entry into the fasted state in a test subject. This data would be essential in deriving a conclusion. Simply speaking, you are going to be consuming a significant number of calories in a relatively short time frame. Ensure you allow yourself ample time to consume what you require while fasting for as long as you can to achieve maximum effect.

Structuring Meals

This is another very subjective topic. After determining what to eat and in which quantities, the next step is to look at how you wish to consume those foods. Meaning, how many meals you would like to eat and the optimal interval between them. Myself included, many proponents of IF choose to break the fast with a significantly larger meal than the others to follow in the day. This may range from 40% to 60% of total intake. This is noticeably more effective when consumed after a fasted training session (we'll be discussing that in depth later on). While not necessarily a recommendation to all, this is another key hack to the method overall.

Otherwise, many find the large meal sits well and satisfies. 800 calories is a fair amount of nutrition in whichever form it may come (an example of this is shown on page __). Suppose you have a TDEE of 2,400cal per day. You would be able to eat two more of those sizable meals each day if you planned a 3-meal schedule. If tapering from a larger breakfast, they may be relatively smaller albeit close in size. Often still quite a stomach's worth.More often than not, folks looking to lose weight are restricting portion size in traditional diets. This is often done as a necessity to creating a caloric deficit. If you enjoy grazing on food and consuming smaller portions, by all means do so. Some may choose a feeding window of 6 hours and consume one meal each hour, totalling 6. Using the above example of a 2,400cal TDEE, said person would be taking in 400 calories at each feeding. This is still a fair number of calories, especially consumed so frequently. This is somewhat an extreme example. However, it highlights the scope of your flexibility within this window. The beauty of the IF method is that you have greater freedom when 'spending' your daily calorie number. Ironically, some clients in the past determined to lose weight have had a hard time eating *enough* by day's end, rather than struggle with eating *too much*. Not a bad problem to have.

Alternate Methods

Method	Description
ADF (Alternate Day Fasting)	24 hours fed; 24 hours fasted (repeat)
5/2 Method	5 concurrent days fed; 2 concurrent days fasted
Eat Stop Eat (by Brad Pilon)	48 hours fed; 24 hours fasted (repeat)
Warrior Diet	Consume only 1 meal per day, everyday

This table highlights alternative methods of intermittent fasting. Intermittent fasting (as we have discussed it thus far) would be defined as Time Restricted Feeding (TRF) for the sake of this study. Alternate Day Fasting (ADF), Alternate Day Modified Fasting (ADMF), and Periodic Feeding (PF) are some other increasingly popular variations of the IF method. These have gained popularity in recent times and thus, have been subjected to far fewer studies than traditional (16:8) style fasting. With a limited amount of scientific data or anecdotal evidence available, a conclusion cannot yet be made regarding which method is most effective.

Many experts in the field suggest that each method may hold its own unique positive and negative traits. For example, the ADF method calls for a full 24-hour fast every second day. Autophagy science tells us that the longer or more frequently we subject ourselves to the 'deprived' state, the greater its effects will be overall. It is speculated that this method may be superior to the (16:8) method with regards to autophagy alone. It's a simple matter of math. However, 3-4 full-day fasts per week may not be feasible for an athlete or someone working an intense labour job. They may require caloric intake daily in order to reserve enough glycogen to perform their activities. If one of the alternate methods sounds more appealing to you than traditional IF, give it a try. They operate on the same principles, utilizing the same science to leverage the body for process improvements. All of the content covered within this book will provide you with enough information to get started with IF, ADF, ADMF, or PF. The next chapter will go into details on how to figure out your individual energy requirement, specific to you.

Your Personal Intake

Now it's time to get a bit personal. We're going to dive into the calculations required to determine your daily caloric requirements. This number will be your baseline- it will be raised and lowered as necessary in order to inch closer to your ultimate goal. This will be discussed more in depth later in the chapter.

There are many ways to estimate your recommended calorie intake, but one of the most accurate is a TDEE calculation. TDEE stands for *Total Daily Energy Expenditure.* In essence, it is the number of calories required in order to support the processes of your body for one entire day at rest. As genders, weights, heights, and body fat percentages vary greatly from person to person, this calculation is specific to you. Excluding mathematical anomalies, no two numbers will be *exactly* the same.

There are a few different methods of arriving at this number. The **Katch McArdle, Cunningham**, and **Harris Benedict** are other popular equations that may be used for the same purpose. While these have been used for quite some time, they are not the most accurate methods of calculation on account of missing a few variables such as age, which does play a considerable role in metabolism (and therefore energy requirements). Please appreciate that no calculation will be absolutely correct, each and every single day. There is an expected +/- tolerance. By selecting the equation that has been studied to have the lowest variance, we stand the best chance of having our numbers balance out over multi-day, weekly, and monthly periods. Sadly, there isn't any way to extract the data from your body (so to speak) in order to measure the daily actual usage vs. consumed usage vs. planned usage. However, just like currency rounding, the assumption is that the numbers will balance out over time with a large enough sample size. For this reason, the TDEE equation we will be using is the **Mifflin-St. Jeor Equation**. It was developed in 1990 and has stood the test of time, being validated by more than 10+ studies across universities and medical journals alike. It provides the highest accuracy rate as well as the lowest overall variance in the subjects.

According to the *American Dietetic Association*, it's the most accurate equation for calculating actual resting energy expenditure to within +/- 10%.

TDEE Formula for Females

Step 1. Calculate BMR *(Basal Metabolic Rate; calories required to support bodily functions at rest)*

BMR = ([Height in Centimeters] x 6.25) + ([Weight in Kilograms] x 9.99) – ([Age] x 4.92) – (161).

Note: [Height in Centimeters = Height in Inches x 2.54]
[Weight in Kilograms = Weight in Pounds x 2.2]

Step 2. Calculate TDEE *(Total Daily Energy Expenditure)*

TDEE = BMR x (Activity Level Factor)

Activity Level Factor Chart

Level	Factor (1.x)	Description
Sedentary	1.1	Little exercise, sedentary job, low impact
Lightly Active	1.275	Light exercise/sports/activity 1-3x per week, sedentary job
Moderately Active	1.35	Moderate exercise/sports/activity 3-5x per week, slightly active job
Very Active	1.525	Heavy exercise/sports/activity 6-7x per week, active job

TDEE Formula for Males

Step 1. Calculate BMR *(Basal Metabolic Rate; calories required to support bodily functions at rest)*

BMR = ([Height in Centimeters] x 6.25) + ([Weight in Kilograms] x 9.99) – ([Age] x 4.92) – (161).

Note: [Height in Centimeters = Height in Inches x 2.54]
[Weight in Kilograms = Weight in Pounds x 2.2]

Step 2. Calculate TDEE *(Total Daily Energy Expenditure)*

TDEE = BMR x (Activity Level Factor)

Activity Level Factor Chart

Level	Factor (1.x)	Description
Sedentary	1.2	Little exercise, sedentary job, low impact
Lightly Active	1.375	Light exercise/sports/activity 1-3x per week, sedentary job
Moderately Active	1.55	Moderate exercise/sports/activity 3-5x per week, slightly active job
Very Active	1.725	Heavy exercise/sports/activity 6-7x per week, active job

Extremely Active	1.9	Very heavy exercise/sports/activity 7-10x per week, physical job

It is very common for people to over-estimate their activity levels. After all, the prospect of being able to consume more food each day is cause for celebration for many (admittedly, myself included at times). For optimum weight loss results, you should select your minimum weekly activity level, rather than your maximum or average. This goes in reverse for those trying to gain weight. The goal here is to err on the side of caution, in whichever direction you wish to travel. This would mean that a person looking to lose weight should use the low estimate of their activity level, while someone looking to gain weight might be better off using the high estimate.

Macronutrients

While the macronutrient composition of your diet may
not directly influence fat loss, it can affect your ability to
adhere to a reduced-calorie diet. To increase your chances
of success on a reduced-calorie diet, individualize your
macronutrient ratio based on your preferences and health.
For example, people with type 2 diabetes may find it easier to control their blood sugars on a low-carb rather than
a high-carb diet. Those engaging in high-energy sports may
require a higher amount of carbs to maintain energy levels
when playing or practicing. Conversely, otherwise healthy
people may find they're less hungry on a high-fat, low-carb
diet, and that it's easier to follow compared to a low-fat,
high-carb diet. However, diets that emphasize a high intake of one macronutrient (like fats) and low intakes of another (like carbs) are not for everyone. In any case, choose
the diet that best fits your lifestyle and preferences. This
may take some trial and error. Ultimately, the time invest-
ment in this is more than worth it when you consider how
pivotal these calulations are to your goals.

The Acceptable Macronutrient Distribution Ranges
(AMDR) set forth by the Institute of Medicine of the National Academies recommend consuming;

45–65% of their calories from carbs
20–35% of their calories from fats

10–35% of their calories from proteins

The body uses these basic units to build substances it needs for growth, maintenance, and activity (including other carbohydrates, proteins, and fats). It's important to note that, by definition, a calorie is a calorie. Be it fat, protein, carbs, or alcohol, 1 calorie = 4.2 joules of energy.
While equal with regard to the energy they provide, the function of these nutrients varies greatly.

Proteins contain amino acids, vital to repairing tissues of all types in the body. The body uses considerable protein when say, healing a laceration or creating new muscle tissue. Protein is not a key source of energy like fat and carbs are. Rather, it is akin to bricks in the scope of home building. Proteins are the bricks- the raw materials necessary to construct the house. Fats and carbs, while fundamentally different, provide the energy to make the project happen. Compare these to the workers building said house.

Note that those engaging in heavy physical labour, training, or weightlifting, will require significantly more protein than someone who is more sedentary.

Fats are the most calorically dense macronutrient, with one gram containing 9cal versus protein and carbs which each contain 4cal per gram. Others, called essential fatty acids, cannot be synthesized and must be consumed in the diet. The essential fatty acids make up about 7% of the fat consumed in a normal diet and about 3% of total calories (about 8 grams). They include linoleic acid and linolenic acid, which are present in certain vegetable oils. Fats in groups such as Omega-3 and Omega-6 contain nutrients essential for brain function and development.

Carbohydrates are used mainly for energy. They are converted into glycogen and stored in the liver and muscles for later use. They are the fastest to digest and the most rapidly available energy source for the body. The quickness at which these create usable energy depends on how highly glycemic they are (low glycemic carbohydrates take much longer to be digested than high glycemic carbs). Some examples of low glycemic foods would be whole grains, sweet potatoes, and brown rice. On the high glycemic side of the index simple sugars, refined syrups, and sweets. The amount of carbohydrates one requires should be gauged upon activity level, as their sole purpose is providing fuel.

These are just brief descriptions of the macronutrients. I recommend doing a little bit more research into these to better educate yourself on the systems of the body and how your food choices affect them. While vitally important information, it falls well beyond the scope of this book.

Calorie Cycling

Following the principles mentioned up to this point as they are presented will undoubtedly be effective. You will be able to achieve great success in your journey regardless of your choosing to opt in to this piece of the puzzle.

To truly weaponize your fat burn and muscle gain arsenal, calorie cycling is the way to go.

Put simply, it is the practice of alternating lower and higher caloric days in accordance with your resting and training days. The purpose of this is to provide your body with more nutrition as it is demanded (post-training), and less when the requirements aren't as high (rest days).

Week-to-week, you will be consuming the same number of calories as you would be when following the standard method. They are just allotted differently over the 7-day period. While this concept does prove effective when bulking or maintaining your weight, it is most optimal when used for the purpose of burning fat. When burning fat, you must be operating in a caloric deficit. As mentioned before, this entails eating less calories each day than your body requires. When the body is in a sustained deficit, it is breaking down fat for energy and muscle for essential amino acids. No matter the goal or the amount carried, muscle is essential to the body. Its functions are endless, but it plays a crucial role in metabolism as well. Muscle contains active mitochondria (cells) that require a significant amount of energy. The more muscle one has, the more baseline calories they require in order to do a given task. For example, two friends go for a jog. Let's call them Tom & Jerry. They are both the same height and weight, and they jog the same distance. Tom's body is 20%

fat and 80% lean tissue, while Jerry is 10% fat and 90% lean tissue. The extra 10% of lean tissue that Jerry has will ultimately require more energy to complete the same run. In addition, a greater taxing of said tissue will also require more caloric intake throughout the period of recovery. Coming back to the original point, it is not advantageous in any way to lose muscle tissue. Calorie cycling puts one in the best position to avoid such atrophy (muscle loss) as the muscles exercised during training will be replenished and refueled in full. On the other hand, the body is able to tap into its stored fat more than normal during rest days since less food is being consumed and introduced into the bloodstream. Low-impact activities done at a fairly low heart rate will not create the need for amino acids to be derived from your precious muscles, while you will be able to tap into fat stores much more easily.

This is the true beauty of caloric cycling.

Consider the following example.

Suppose my TDEE is 2,500cal per day at baseline.
Let's say my goal is to lose 1lb per week (500cal deficit per day).
My daily intake would then be 2,000cal per day, or 14,000 for the week.
I train three days out of the week and rest for four.

Monday (Train).............2,500cal
Tuesday (Rest)................1,500cal
Wednesday (Train)........2,500cal
Thursday (Rest)..............1,500cal
Friday (Train)................2,500cal
Saturday (Rest)...............1,500cal
Sunday (Rest).................2,000cal

With some simple addition, it is clear that the goal of 14,000cal per week is met in the example. Note that Sunday does not follow the typical 1,500 for a rest day. This is shown to balance the numbers over the week. Eating the standard 1,500 calories would result in a greater deficit over the 7-day span. Please note that your optimal deficit depends largely on how much fat you carry. Those with much excess can stand to operate on lower intake, as their bodies have progressively been storing calories for such a point in time. The leaner you become, the more your body will resist fat loss. This happens for biological reasons. The body senses that less and less nutrition is coming in consistently and strives to store all that it can in case the deficit grows larger or food suddenly stops becoming available. Keep in mind that we know our ultimate plan in the mind, but the body acts more instinctively.

A Look at Food Selection

I understand that the contents of the last chapter may be cause for excitement if your dieting strategy has been very selective up to this point. I remember the joy I felt when I was able to expand my horizons beyond chicken, brown rice, and vegetables. Free to attend restaurants and outings with friends as I pleased. The complete freedom with food choices really will do wonders for your mindset with regard to long-term goal setting and staying the course overall. It feels far more sustainable; it begins to feel like

more of a lifestyle choice and less of an implied struggle. I would like to take this time to make a very clear distinction. Eating to improve health, and eating to achieve a weight or physique goal, are not married concepts. Refer to the macronutrients concept and TDEE calculations we went over in a previous chapter. It is possible for anyone to eat mainly unwholesome foods and become a lean, ripped, performance machine. What's ultimately required is calculating their necessary caloric intake and adjusting their actual intake in accordance to their goal. Likewise, someone who is eating a plethora of healthy foods in excess of their necessary intake over time *will* gain fat. Recall that fat is stored energy from our last chapter. Sadly, the body does not store 'better quality' fat if the foods consumed are micronutrient dense. Again, this goes against many long-held beliefs, yet the science is there. This does not just apply to intermittent fasting either, it holds true no matter how often you feed or fast. 2 hours, 8 hours, 16 hours- the timing is not a factor when considering this principle. With that being said, the optimal solution is to *consume the required number of calories from natural sources that provide the highest amount of macronutrients.* Understanding that this point is something of an equilibrium- constantly shifting and rarely steady- all we must do is make the best available choice at the time. Every time. We may not ever have a perfect day, but we understand this going in. The freedom to know that you could fall back on a full daily intake's worth of Burger King and not lose any momentum on the ride to your goal will give you an odd sense of motivation to try and eat as best you can. I know it may sound highly contrary, but it's the way things seem to go for those who have adopted the model and felt it worked for them. The mind often works in mysterious ways.

Consider the following example.

The McDonald's Scenario

You take a trip to your local McDonald's and order yourself 2 McDouble™ sandwiches.

The calorie total for **(2) McDoubles** in Toronto, Ontario, Canada is **740cal.**

This is comprised of 42(g) protein, 34(g) fat [16g saturated], and 68(g) carbohydrates.

This delicious burger duo will also net you 120mg of cholesterol (38% Recommended Daily Intake), 1720mg of sodium (72% of R.D.I), and 14g of sugar.

Micronutrient wise, you'll be looking at 6% and 2% of your R.D.I for Vitamin A and C, respectively.

Now, say, you've decided to stay in the next night and cook a meal yourself. For the sake of this example, you're trying to hit the same macronutrient totals as you did the night previous at the Golden Arches.

You cook a delicious meal featuring a cup of diced, seasoned chicken as the main feature. It is paired with 2 cups of quinoa and grilled asparagus with an olive oil drizzle. The macronutrient totals for this meal are 46(g) protein, 34(g) fat, and 64(g) carbohydrates.

While not exactly identical, the two examples are within +/- 5% of each other. In effect, they fare the same by way of caloric intake and macronutrient composition.

The key difference is that the second meal boasts Vitamins A, B, B6, C, and D. Substantial amounts of magnesium and potassium, with little sodium (7% of R.D.I compared to 72%). A good mix of these three is essential to balancing electrolytes. Vitamin B_{12}, also known as cobalamin, is a water-soluble vitamin that is involved in the metabolism of every cell of the human body- it is present in sufficient quantity (15%). Last but not least, there is plentiful polyunsaturated and monounsaturated fat content- 4.98g and 22.23g respectively. These two are referred to as 'essential fats'. In essence, they help with everything from brain function (coordination, memory, recall, etc.) to lowering risk of heart disease and type 2 diabetes.

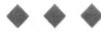

You want those micronutrients. You *need* them.

Your body will operate all of its millions of processes smoother, armed with the building blocks and steady energy to do so. You will feel better. Your skin will look better. You will feel sharper mentally. More energetic. Your body will certainly appreciate it. After all, the difference is akin to premium 93 Octane fuel vs a low quality, poorly filtered 85. Your vehicle (your body) will still run. The numbers are there. The gas is in the tank. Wouldn't you rather choose the premium? Why not be at your best?

To sum it up, I hope you are able to come to terms with this concept. Relieve your mind from the tunnel vision of the standard weight loss diets. Restricting your feeding windows is enough on you already. Enjoy. Indulge. Monitor your intake. Stay on track with your numbers.

Just remember, always strive to make the choices that will have you waking up your best in the morning. If you need a good indulgence to get back on track, do it. If you've been sluggish lately and require more nutrient dense foods, eat them. Do what's best for your mental and physical state as their needs change and adapt. You're in control.

Supplements

There has been little research done on common nutritional supplements and their effects on fasting. Vitamin supplements, pre-workout supplements, post-workout supplements- there are many different categories, let alone individual proprietary blends and combinations.

Things such as 0-calorie Branched Chain Amino Acid (BCAA) drink mixes, 0-calorie pre-workout supplements, vitamin tablets, and pharmaceuticals may be consumed during the fasting period. They have not been observed to cause any disruption to the processes that be.

Protein supplements (bars, shakes, smoothies), intra-workout carbohydrate solutions, and many fibre supplements are best suited for the feeding window. They may otherwise take you out of the fasted state before you've schedule yourself to do so. The general rule of thumb to follow with supplements is to *consume only 0-calorie supplements during your fast, opting for calorie-containing supplements during the fasting period.* If you are unsure whether or not a supplement contains calories, check the product's packaging. If this information is unavailable on the packaging, contact the manufacturer. By law (in most of North America at least), food and supplement producers are legally required to disclose the ingredients and nutritional information pertaining to their product.

Substance Use & Fasting

Given the nature of the method as scheduled consumption of food and beverage, questions often arise regarding alcohol's effects on fasting (and that of other substances as well). It is important to first separate alcohol from other drugs on account of alcohol containing calories.

Alcohol

In the *Personal Intake* chapter, we talked about macronutrient profiles and their individual caloric makeup per gram. Recall that proteins and carbohydrates carry 4cal per gram, while fat carries 9. Nestled in the middle of these two figures is alcohol, netting a cool 7.1cal per gram. The **Thermic Effect of Food (TEF)** sees the real value of alcohol drop to roughly 5.7cal per gram. This metric measures the amount of energy expenditure above the basal metabolic rate due to the cost of processing food for use and storage. A quick example to highlight this concept would be a small business- they take in '7cals' of revenue, but after expense spending, net income is '5.7cals'. The business only retains the 5.7 although it grossed the full 7.

This is an important concept to dieting- its full breadth, however, is beyond the scope of this book.

As we now know, consumption of calories during the fasting period will break said fast upon entry into the bloodstream. Quite simply, this means no alcohol during your fast. You intake it, you break it. Studies have consistently shown that moderate drinkers tend to live longer than non-drinkers. This can be mainly attributed to a lowered risk of cardiovascular disease. However, alcohol also contributes to a healthier and disease-free life by protecting against Alzheimer's disease, metabolic syndrome, rheumatoid arthritis, the common cold, different types of cancers, and a host of other cardiovascular illnesses common in Western society. It has also been proven to reduce the insulin-hypertension relationship that plays a major role in diabetes and insulin sensitivity overall. The *Hisayama study* highlights this correlation.

The fitness and health industry often shuns alcohol on account of its testosterone-dampening effects. These claims are often exaggerated. A 3-week study that had its subjects consume 3 beers per day for 3 weeks observed only a 6.8% reduction in testosterone for males and 0% for women. The effect of alcohol on muscle protein synthesis is unknown in normal human subjects. It is not unlikely to assume that a negative effect exists, but it is very unlikely that it is of such a profound magnitude purported in fitness literature.

The bottom line is, humans have enjoyed alcohol for entire millennia. It does not appear to be going away anytime soon. Enjoy it. Have a few drinks with your coworkers after work or take in a nice glass of wine with your spouse. Just be cautious of your fasting window. Remember, even clear spirits with no chaser contain at least an effective 5.7cal per gram. Factor the calories you consume from drinking into your daily totals and live a little!

Illicit Substances

With regard to other drugs (running the gamut from marijuana to crystal methamphetamine), the conversation is a bit different as these do not directly affect your fast. They do not contain calories and no recreational drug available today is metabolized by the body to produce energy via fatty acids, glucose, amino acids, or ethanol. Consumption of substances other than alcohol during your fast will not halt it on their own accord.

An important distinction to make is the *indirect* effects of substance use on one's ability to adhere to their regime. Recreational substances have impacts on the mind by definition and by purpose. These effects vary greatly between people- tolerance, age, experience, height, weight, gender will all play a role in how one's mind processes the substance in question. Let's look at marijuana for example. New and inexperienced smokers are likely to be hit with a strong wave of sedation, a great impulse to consume food ('munchies', colloquially), and a general sense of euphoria and disorientation. They may feel less inhibitions and take more risks. These could prove themselves as great difficulties to someone looking to remain steadfast on intermittent fasting. The temptation of the chip bag may be all too great. Likewise, an experienced habitual smoker becomes immune to these effects or feels them significantly less. In some cases, smokers exhibit the opposite of those effects over the long term. I have seen many folks who have a duller appetite with marijuana and seem far more energetic and talkative than when sober. It is very much a subjective conversation. This paradox can be seen across users of common recreational drugs, from cocaine to opiates.

There is no catch-all or verified information I could provide on this topic. It is a personal issue that only you will know how to approach. The key take-away point is that you may enjoy some light use while fasting but be honest with yourself. Always be reminded of your ultimate goals, but don't be afraid to enjoy life in the interim.

Smoking & Fasting

If you're a smoker looking to dive into the world of IF, I've got some bad news and I've got some good news. The bad news is that, as per the *World Health Organization*, tobacco kills more than 7 million people worldwide on an annual basis. It is certainly a habit that drains you of your resources here on earth- health, wealth, and time. I'm sure you've received countless lectures on this in the past. I am not here to provide another.

The good news is that smoking bears no outright impact on your fasting windows, feeding times, or ability to be successful in your goals. Cigarettes, vaporizers, snuff- whichever product you fancy, they do not contain calories nor stoke the fire on metabolic processes that may throw off your progress. With that being said, smoking does affect some of the essential processes in the body that go beyond breathing. When tobacco smoke is inhaled, it forms carbon monoxide and binds with hemoglobin to traverse through the blood stream. When this occurs, oxygen levels become depleted in the bloodstream. Oxygen is used in this fashion to produce energy within the body. Naturally, the less oxygen your cells are able to distribute throughout the body, the less efficient it will be with everything from recycling lactic acid to delivering nutrients to your muscles following training.

Please note that this is a hindrance to your *efficiency*, and not your *ability*. You are still completely capable of reaching whatever goal you wish to accomplish via IF, while being a smoker. It will just be harder on your body internally to complete these processes day after day.

Another study I would like to highlight relates more specifically to smoking while fasting. This experiment indicated that when studying smokers in both "fed" and "fasted" control groups, the blood level carbon monoxide was significantly higher in the fasted group versus the fed group (30.3ppm to 28.1ppm, respectively).

This information tells us that smoking during the fast will result in higher levels of carbon monoxide circulation than if consumption were to occur during the fed state. This results in lower levels of oxygen and hemoglobin, essential for carrying nutrients and glycogen throughout the body. Science has not yet come out with answers to the prolonged effects of smoking while fasting intermittently. Presumably, smoking will not result in any greater benefit when compared with non-smoking due to the health risks it poses to the body overall. It's best to err on the side of caution and make efforts to reduce consumption.

We can conclude that smoking during your fasting window will result in less oxygen being transmitted and more free radicals flowing throughout your body. It would then follow that, scientifically, it is less detrimental to smoke during the feeding window. While I understand this habit may be harder to schedule due to its addictive and habit-forming nature, these are just the facts. Smoking will not break your fast- it may even assist in suppressing appetite. It will, however, eventually break the bank and damage your respiratory system. I would be remiss if I didn't communicate these facts objectively.

Fasted Training

By now, I'm sure the concepts of fasted-state and fed-state are clear as day. We leverage these two periods for different reasons in order to make the most efficient use of our energy and calories.

Standard industry advice would tell you to consume food or beverage prior to training in order to fuel your workout and provide energy to your body. As we now know, the body retains glucose in the muscles as energy for intense activity on more of a daily cycle than an hourly one. If following IF principles, you will have taken in a fair excess of carbohydrates that will be made available to you during your next workout. The body likes to be efficient, therefore it will utilize any and all calories available in the digestion system before having to break down its reserves (fat & glucose). Without the presence of said calories, the body is able to tap directly into these stores. Following the session, the fast is broken. The initial load of calories is processed at a time when the body is starving for nutrients and its ability to partition is at its peak. With a greater demand for calories present, your body is far less likely to store these as fat since they need to be used once consumed. The concept of fasted training is essentially twofold;

As you train, your body breaks down glucose and oxidizes

(burns) fat to procure the calories necessary to facilitate the efforts. In turn, you perform more *direct* fat burning.

On the flip side, the post-training feed occurs when your body is in its most depleted state, ready to utilize your intake to repair, rebuild, and refresh.

A recent study shows fasted training affects the post-workout anabolic response to weight training more favorably than fed-state training. This study is very interesting to say the least, since it lends scientific support to explain the beneficial effects from both fasted-training and Leangains-style intermittent fasting. Let me give you the lowdown on this study in layman's terms. Weight training activates enzymes and switches on genes that up regulates protein synthesis in muscles. Out of these signalling mechanisms, the phosphorylation, "activity" plainly speaking, of p70s6 kinase may serve as an indicator of muscle growth, along with other myogenic transcription factors. Myogenic meaning from within the muscle. Nutrition no doubt affects the myogenic signaling mechanisms, but it's

still not fully understood to what degree. In this study, subjects were split into two groups that were trained on two occasions separated by three weeks. The three-week rest period between sessions served as a "washout" period, in order to make sure that the prior session didn't interfere with the results obtained during the second test. The workouts were fairly basic whole-body sessions: 3 x 8 in seven movements such as bench press, overhead press, curls and leg press.One of the sessions (F) were performed on an empty stomach after an overnight fast.The other session (B) was performed in the fed state. Subjects were given a breakfast of 722 kcal composed of 85% carbs, 11% protein and 4% fat, and training was initiated 90 minutes after the meal. After the weight training session, both groups rested for 4 hours. At the one- and four-hour marks, muscle biopsies and blood tests were obtained. Participants were also given a recovery drink to sip each hour during the rest period. Results revealed that the F session had twice as high levels of p70s6k in comparison to the B when measured at the one-hour mark post-workout. Other myogenic transcription factors were also higher at this point, though not quite as pronounced as p70s6k. At the four-hour mark, the differences between the two groups had evened out.

Why may fasted training be beneficial for the post-workout anabolic response?

The researchers concluded that "Our results indicate that prior fasting may stimulate the intramyocellular anabolic response to ingestion of a carbohydrate/protein/leucine mixture following a heavy resistance training session." Among other things, increased levels of p70s6k may lead to a faster transport of amino acids into the muscle cell membranes, which should lead to a more rapid and potent anabolic response to post-workout nutrient ingestion. The effects seen on the other myogenic signaling mechanisms could also affect muscle growth through other pathways.

It seems that the increased anabolic activity seen post-workout is a compensatory response to the increased catabolism that occurs during fasted state training. Very interesting. The big question is if there would be a net difference in muscle growth at the end of the day. Training on an empty stomach will cause greater catabolism in the short run, but will it yield greater gains in the long run? Do we make a small sacrifice in order to receive a greater reward? Well, I think we can leverage the results of this study to our benefit and sidestep the negatives if we ask ourselves why, relative to the fasted group, p70s6k and the other myogenic transcription factors were inhibited after a pre-workout meal. Or rather the highly insulinogenic pre-workout meal served in the study — a whopping 153 g high glycemic index carbs. There's no clear answer here, but other studies have suggested that carb intake during an endurance training can blunt the expression of several metabolic genes post-exercise. Insulin may play a role here, for sure.

Another way to think of it is that by providing nutrients to the body, exercise is experienced by the body as less of a stressor compared to fasted-state training. No need to adapt or compensate when all is provided for you. A similar phenomenon can be seen with antioxidant intake, where recent studies show that ingesting antioxidants from supplements weakens the body's own response to deal with free radicals created by training. We are making it easy for the body and that may be a suboptimal way to train.

So, do I suggest everyone start training fasted from now on? Of course not. Remember, it is still not known if the net effect of fasted state training will lead to more favorable results in the long run. Make sure that the great majority of your daily allotment of calories and carbs are ingested in the post-workout period, and not before.

The immediate pre-workout meal should contain no more than a moderate amount of low glycemic index carbs. The exact amount would depend on many factors, total workout volume being the biggest one to consider, but a good guideline for a moderate volume weight training session is approximately 0.6 – 0.8 g carb per kilogram body weight or 0.3 – 0.4 g per pound of body weight. Have this meal 1.5 – 2.5 hours before your training session.

For fasted sessions, ingest 10 g branched chain amino acids (BCAA) shortly prior (5-15 mins) to your training session. This does not count towards the 8-hour feeding window that I advocate post-workout; that starts with your post-workout meal. By ingesting BCAA pre-workout, we can sidestep the increased protein breakdown of fasted training while still reaping the benefits of the increased anabolic response as seen in this study. Not only that, BCAAs actually increase phosphorylation of p70s6k when ingested in the fasted state prior to training. So, by training fasted with BCAA intake prior to sessions, we get a double whammy of increased p70s6k phosphorylation that should create a very favorable environment for muscle growth in the post-workout period.

Longevity & Practicality

The question of longevity is often raised when assessing the long-term effectiveness of intermittent fasting. The idea of sectioning off two thirds of each available day to fast may not seem feasible over a long period of time with regard to social gatherings and planning for events. In fact, the opposite is true. Once you get the hang of your personal fasting techniques, it becomes simple. It becomes a second nature. Most who begin to fast and experience the benefits continue to do so into perpetuity. I know I personally couldn't see myself eating any other way. If not for the benefits, for the simple *convenience*.

Consider the following example.

Suppose you are a fairly social person and you've decided to break your fast each day around lunchtime. This leaves breakfast (or brunch, depending on the time) as the one 'standard' meal that you'll generally be skipping. As social norms go in present day Western society, breakfast is not often a meal that families or organizations sit down for. Throughout chaotic weeks, hectic schedules, and absurd traffic volume, we often fight the good fight to get to our place of work and presume with business as usual. You will likely find that without the need to prepare breakfast or make a pit stop for it, you'll have more time to yourself. However, you choose to use said time is up to you. Once this becomes a habit, you'll likely find that skipping breakfast is in fact more practical than halting your life to consume it.

Fast forward to mid-day. It's now lunchtime and your colleagues have decided to go out to a restaurant for lunch. You've been fasted up to this point and it's time to break the fast. You may usually be skimping on the dishes you'd really like in favor of lower-calorie options. When fasting consistently, your body will be able to partition (digest & disperse in the body) nutrients more effectively. This often results in little to no bloating. I'm sure we are all familiar with the afternoon productivity drop-off that follows a large feast. When fasting, this becomes difficult to achieve. You'd need to eat an absurd amount to be feeling sleepy and groggy to that degree. You'll also be able to enjoy higher-calorie foods. After all, this typically is your largest meal of the day. Maybe you've had a few snacks throughout the day or maybe a beverage of sorts.

Dinner becomes more or less the same as lunch. Depending on your specific daily requirements and intake up to that point, it may be a smaller meal, the same size, or larger. You'll be much freer with your choices and open to a wider range of places and recipes. After this meal, you'll be able to look at what you've eaten today and determine whether or not you have room for some nighttime snacking. Often times you'll find you may have a great deal of net calories available to consume. Many diets advise against night time eating. If your feeding window falls in this timeframe, you've got the clear go ahead to enjoy yourself. Think of it as your reward for fasting through the morning and being more productive. Many find eating at this time of day soothing. Typically, your tasks for the day are complete and you've begun to relax. Maybe you're watching a movie. Maybe you're reading a book. Whatever you're doing, chances are slim to none that you'll be fixated on food you can't have; calories you can't consume. After finishing your last feeding of the day, enjoy some water or possibly tea. You'll be satiated, relaxed, and ready to close the curtain on another good day. Your final hours of the day begin your fast, your sleep furthers it along, and you wake up in the morning to do it all over again.

While results may differ for everyone, these are the most common observations made by those who fast.

Seeming like an improbable and highly unpractical method initially, it becomes clear that intermittent fasting and time restricted feeding may in fact be significantly more practical than traditional dieting. At the very least, it removes the need to worry- even think- about food for 8 more hours each day. Representing 33% of your life over time, this is an impressive gain for anyone. Imagine being a business, instantly able to increase your manufacturing capacity by a third using no more resources than consumed currently. Amazing!

Outro

Well, there you have it. You're ready to start fasting.

I'm sure this all seems too good to be true. It may be down-right unbelievable. I certainly thought so at one time.

The sciences have been responsible for many great discoveries over the millennia. The internet, commercial flight, the telephone- the list goes on and on. During the inception period of these great inventions, they were also looked at with disbelief. Even as positive results became apparent, they remained difficult to comprehend. Eventually, even the biggest skeptic would become unable to scrutinize them. You can't quite reject the idea of the telephone being feasible technology when they are becoming household items. When all your neighbours have clued in, asking why you couldn't see the light earlier.

I believe fasting and time restricted feeding are quite similar in nature. They provide benefits unheard of when dieting the way we have always been conditioned to. It has the potential to dramatically improve our efficiency and quality of life. It is so fundamentally counter-intuitive to what we have always learned about nutrition that many believe it to be a fad or a gimmick. I recall being laughed at many times in my early years with fasting when trying to explain the concepts to others, let alone talk about its benefits. Some of those same people have now began to implement the principles. A few are going a step further and educating others. Please appreciate that I have strictly discussed *proven, studied, verified* effects and benefits of IF in this book.

Science is well underway with examining links to fasting in aiding chemotherapy patients, as well as preventing and treating cancer, and increasing life expectancy. As of now, the results look promising. However, without a larger sample size to draw conclusions from, it remains somewhat speculative. These are just a few of the major findings that researchers are beginning to uncover. It's quite an exciting time to be studying IF and an even more exciting time to get started with it.

I sincerely hope you've enjoyed this book. More importantly, that you've learned this formula and gained valuable insight that you may apply to your life. Please share it with your friends and family. I'm not particularly greedy- I want everyone to be in on this wonderful secret.

One day soon, it will be secret no longer.